Dot Discovery

Dogs

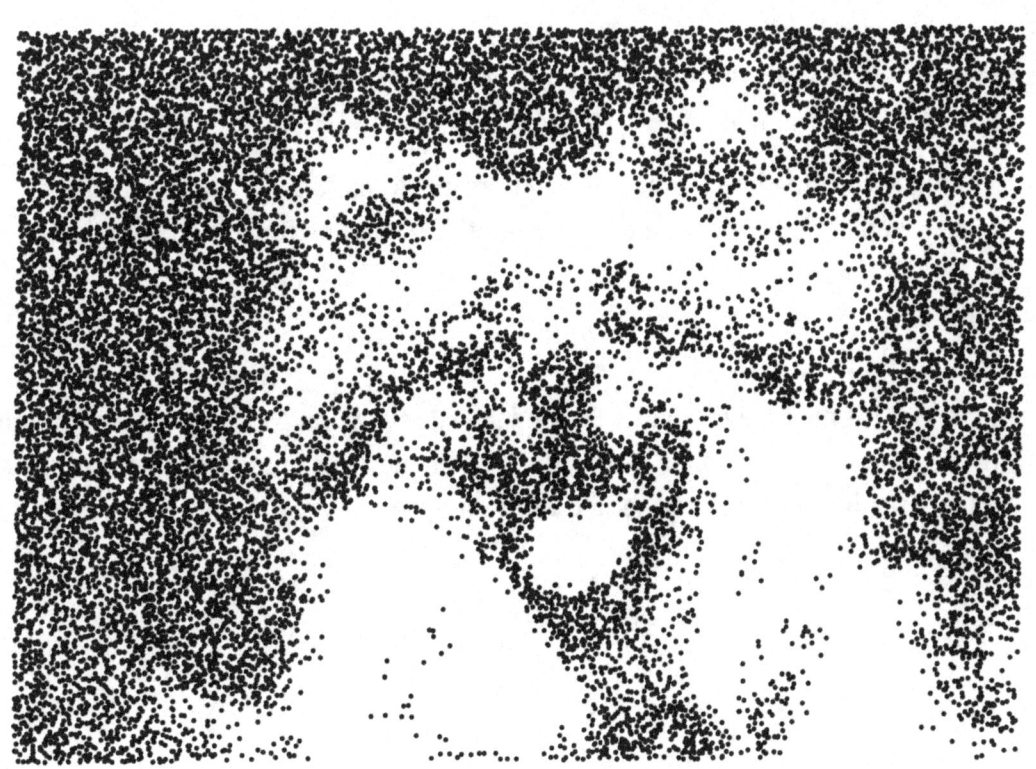

Easy, Stress-free Relaxation by Creating Hand-Drawn Images of Your Favorite Dogs

Adult Coloring Book – Dot Discovery

Dogs

Easy, Stress-free Relaxation by Creating Hand-Drawn Images of Your Favorite Dogs

Get Started Discovering!

Now is the time to take a deep breath and relax. Simply by placing the number of dots in the area specified, an image will appear. By focusing on the dots, you will release stress from the outside world and create lovely hand-drawn pictures.

This book is a unique coloring book. You can use basic black markers, or choose a different color to change things up. Spend a few minutes a day revealing the secret pictures hidden in the pages.

Thanks for your support!

I would love a review, it means a lot to me. Please leave a review on Amazon. Every comment, idea, and compliment is a huge motivation. Reading them helps me create products that suit your desires, and lets customers see how you have benefited from this book.

Dot Discovery

Dot Discovery is a unique and innovative coloring style. Rather that coloring in lines, you place dots whimsically on top of the numbers. Using a medium-sized felt tipped pen or marker, simply stipple over and around the number using the number's amount of dots. If a number says 1, place one dot anywhere around the number. If it says 9, place 9 dots around the number. You should vary where you put the dots and space them all around the number. As you continue with this process, slowly a picture will reveal itself.

This coloring book is fun for both adults and children. We hope you enjoy it! The pages are single sided, so you can remove your finished work and proudly display it. Your friends and family will be amazed at what you have created almost as much as you enjoyed creating it.

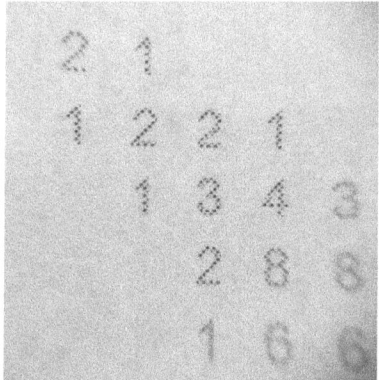

The numbers tell you how many dots to add

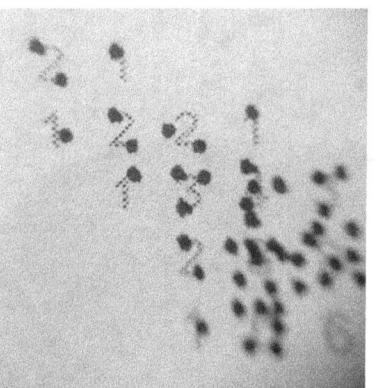

Just add the dots anywhere around the number

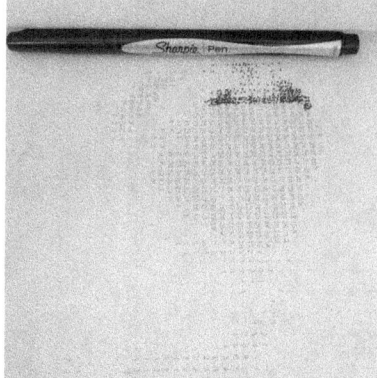

Keep going and before you know it....

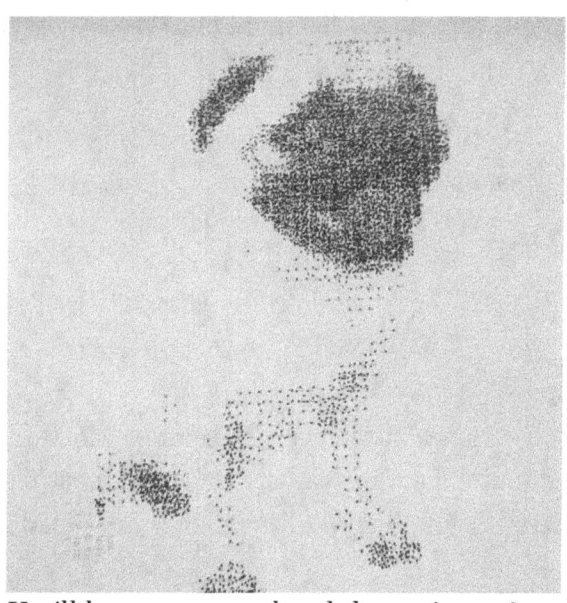

You'll have your own hand-drawn image!

Marker Size & Levels

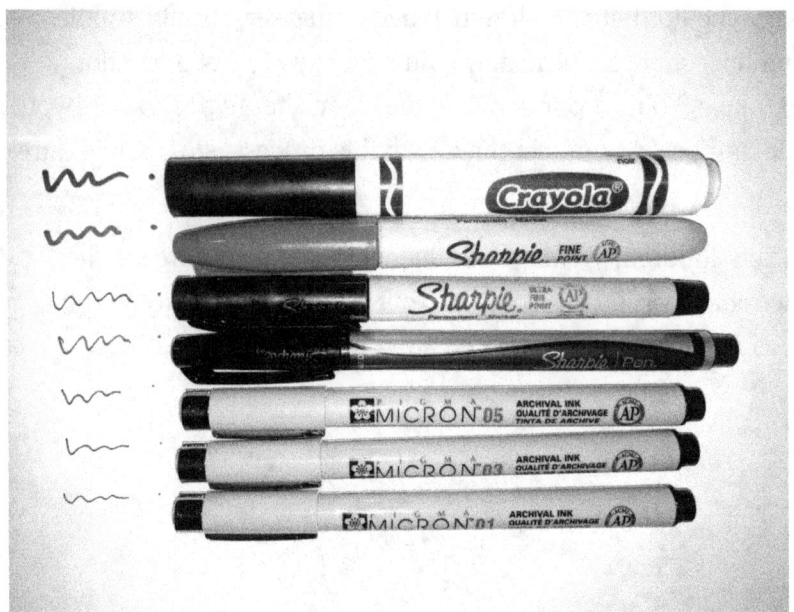

Broadest to finest (top to bottom):

Crayola Classic Broad Line marker
Sharpie Fine Marker
Sharpie Ultra Fine Marker
Sharpie Medium Pen
Pigma Micron .45mm Ink Pen
Pigma Micron .35mm Ink Pen
Pigma Micron .25mm Ink Pen

There are 4 levels of drawings, each sized for different ink pens or markers:

- **Easy** – Crayola Classic Broad Line marker, Crayola Pipsqueak marker, or Sharpie Fine *Marker* is recommended.

- **Intermediate** – Sharpie Fine *Marker*, Crayola Classic Broad Line marker, Crayola Pipsqueak marker is recommended.

- **Advanced** – Sharpie Ultra Fine *Marker* or Sharpie Fine *Pen* (or Sharpie Medium *Pen*) is recommended.

- **Expert** – Pigma Micron Ink Pens .45mm, .35mm, or .25mm recommended.

Note – There is a difference between Sharpie Markers and Sharpie Pens. The pens are black, as seen on the previous page. The markers have a grey barrel. Note that the Sharpie Fine Pen has a finer point than the Sharpie Ultra Fine Marker which is finer than the Sharpie Fine Marker.

Tips

- If you use Sharpie Markers or Pens, you will need to either remove the page or put something under it so that the ink does not bleed through onto the image below.

- For best consistency, always draw on the same surface. A soft surface (such as a magazine) will allow the ink to spread a little more, whereas a hard surface keeps the point slightly smaller.

- Make sure your dots are evenly distributed over the whole number, otherwise there may be darker concentrations in the middle of the number.

- *Have fun!*

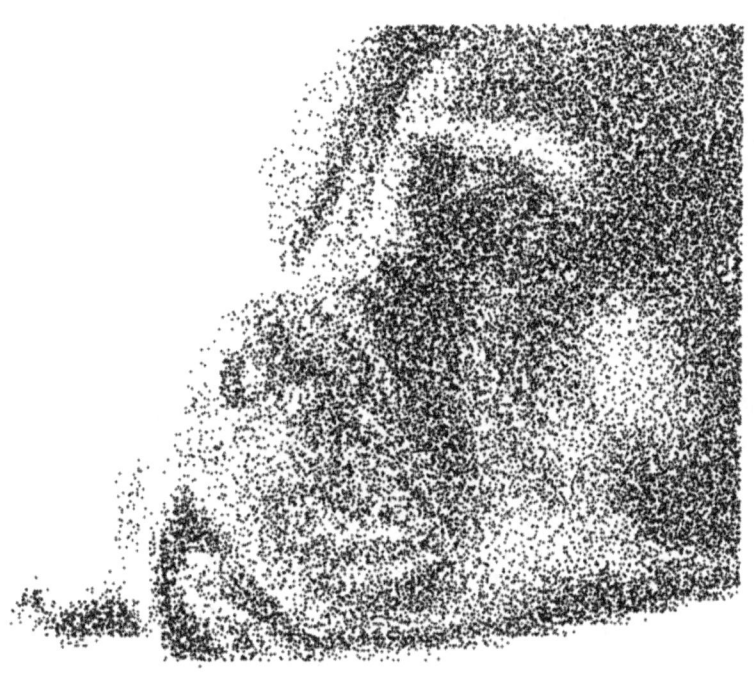

Colorist's Name

_____

Date Started _____

Date Completed _____

Drawings

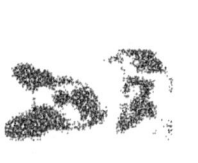

beginner

3636 Dots

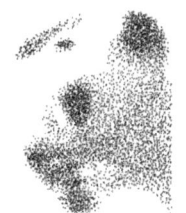

beginner

5536 Dots

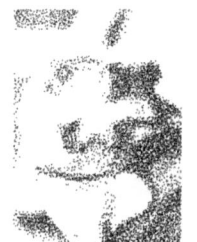

beginner

7306 Dots

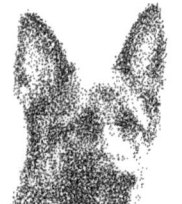

beginner

10058 Dots

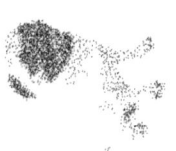

intermediate

2488 Dots

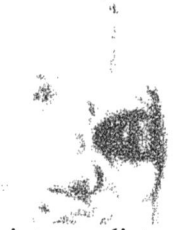

intermediate

3953 Dots

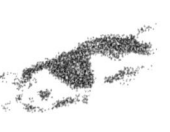

intermediate

2798 Dots

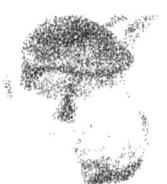

intermediate

4446 Dots

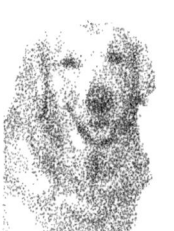

intermediate

7763 Dots

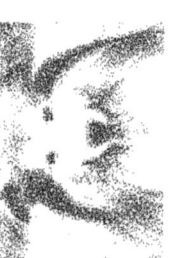

intermediate

9440 Dots

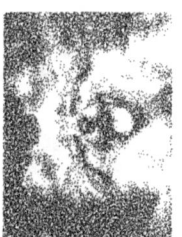

intermediate

20032 Dots

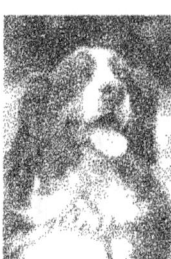

advanced

33345 Dots

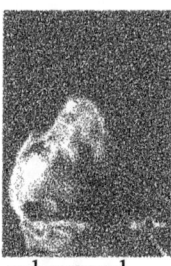

advanced

58990 Dots

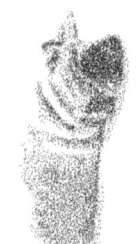

advanced

7868 Dots

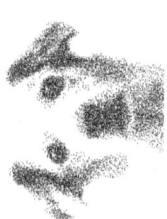

advanced

10512 Dots

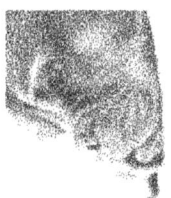

advanced

15027 Dots

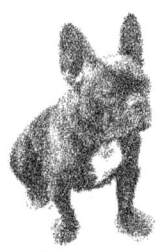

expert

25735 Dots

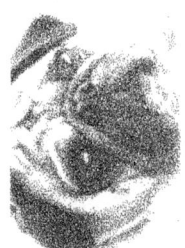

expert

32496 Dots

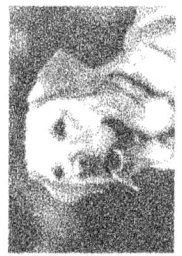

expert

41006 Dots

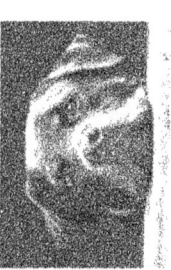

expert

51696 Dots

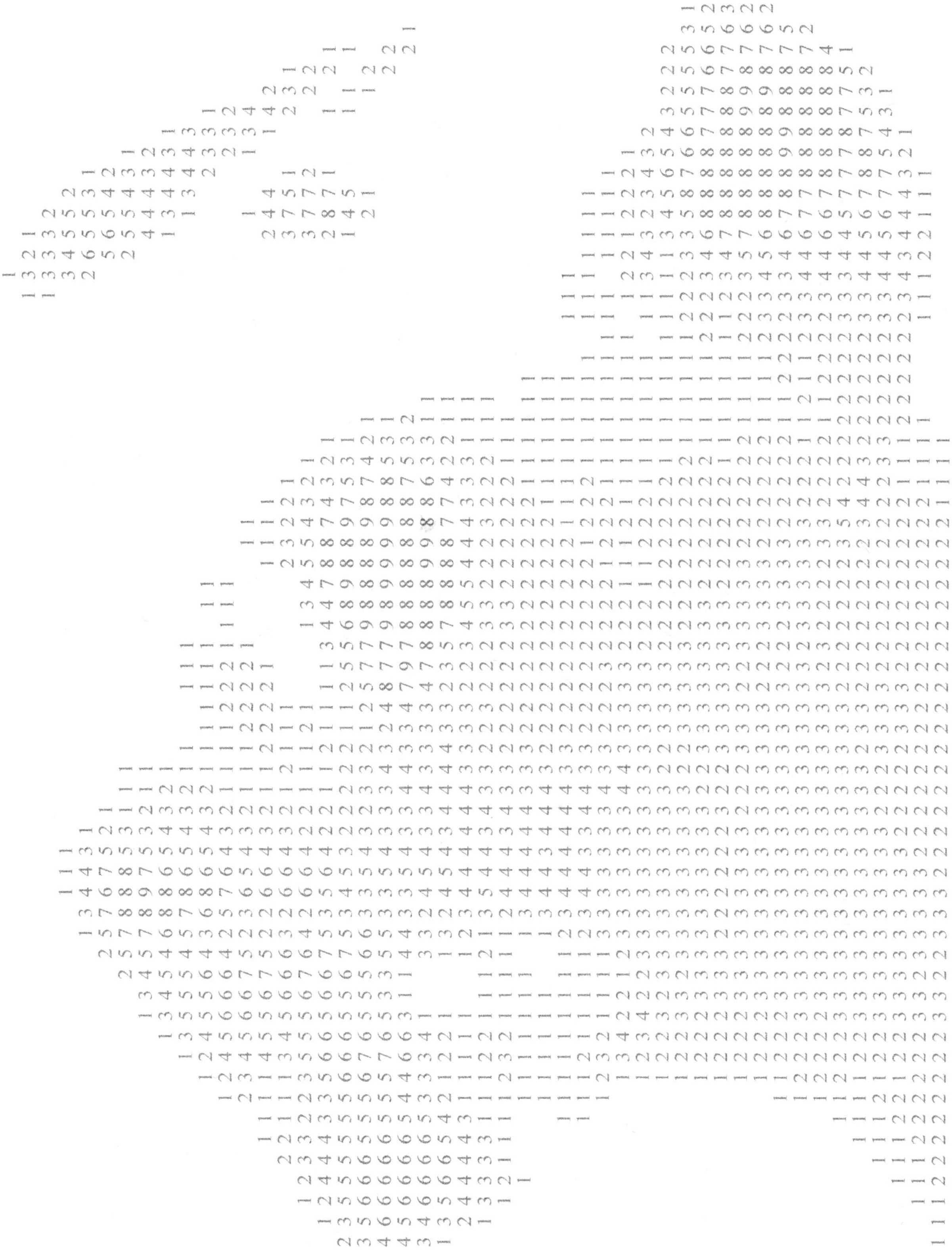

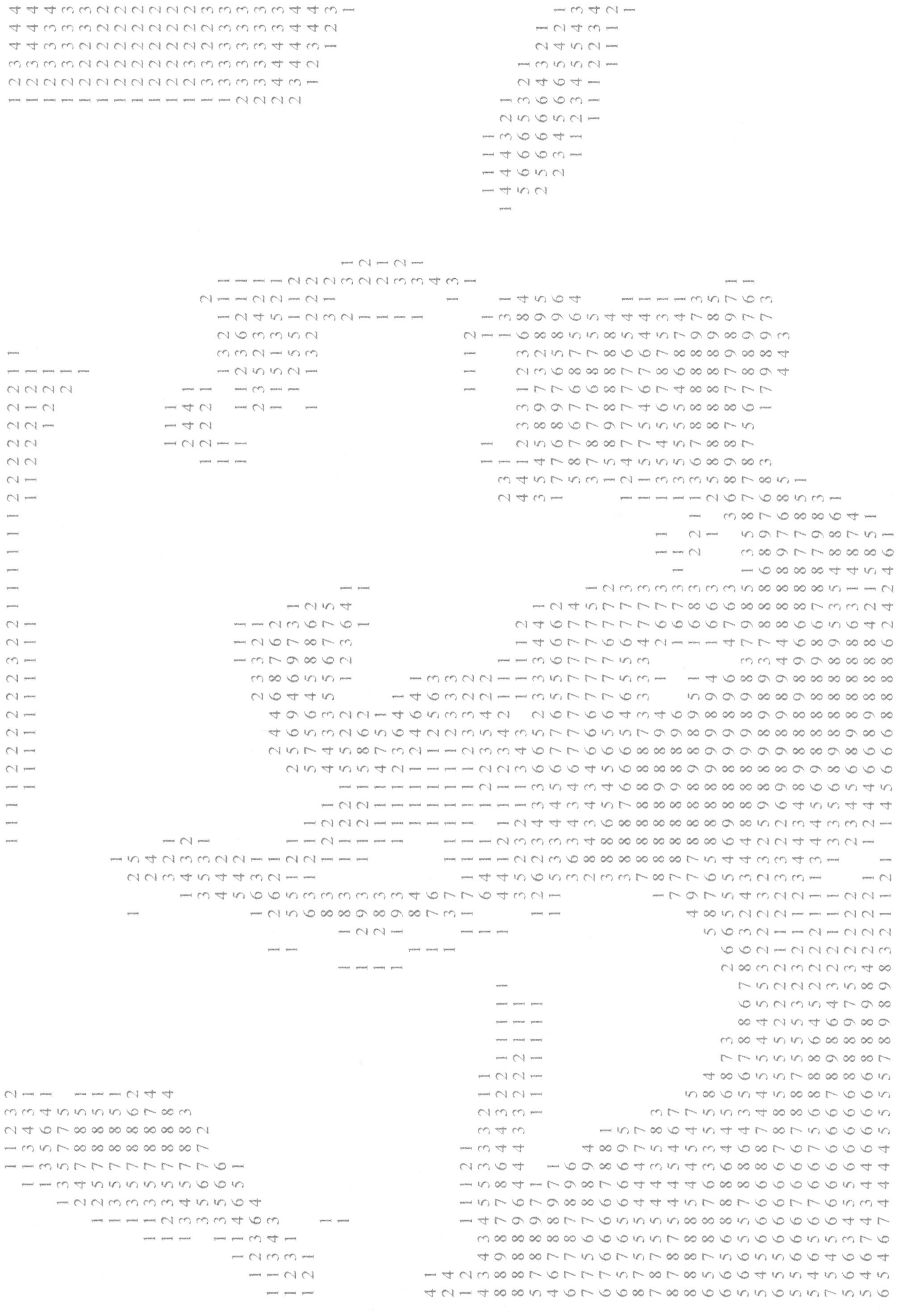

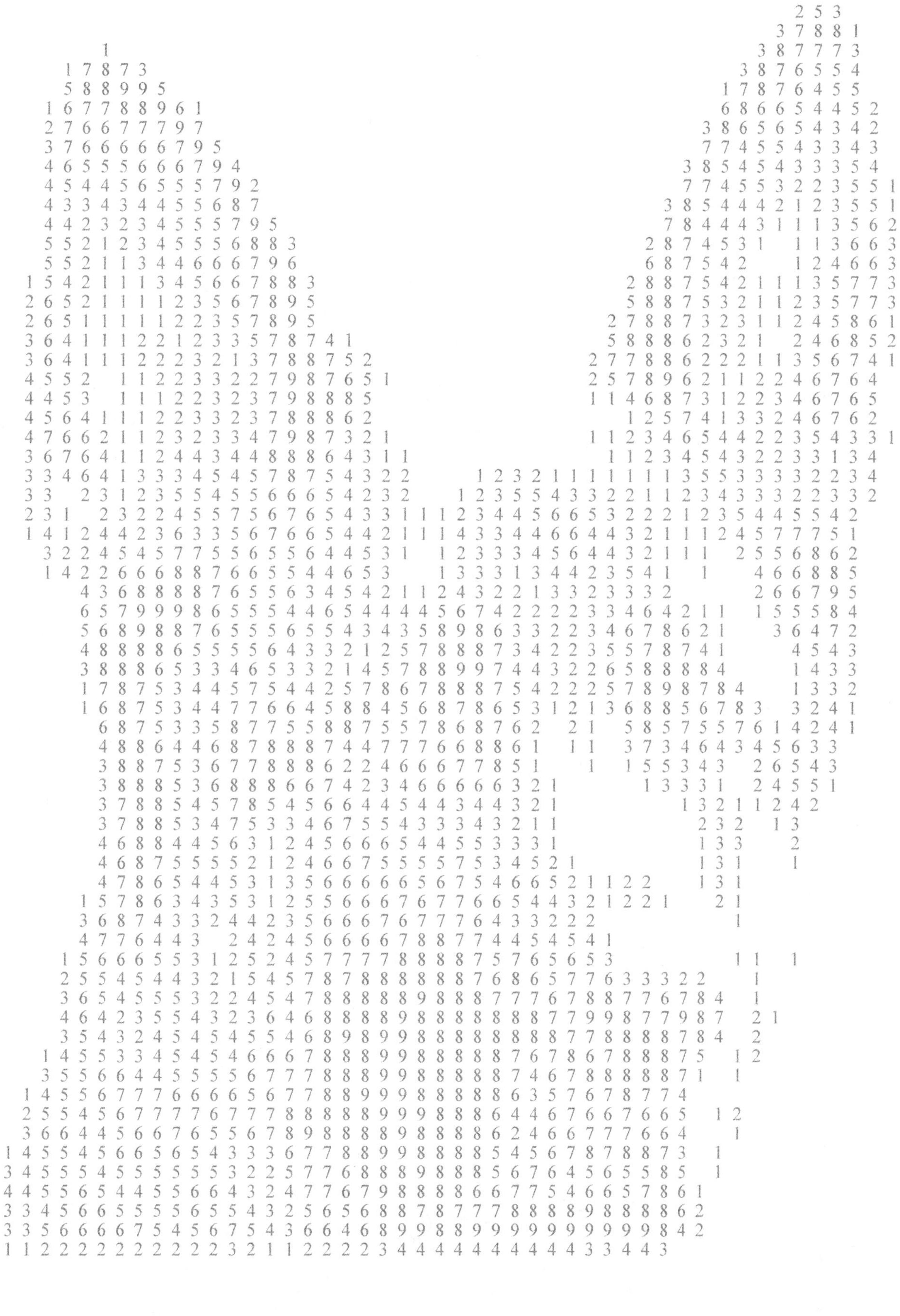

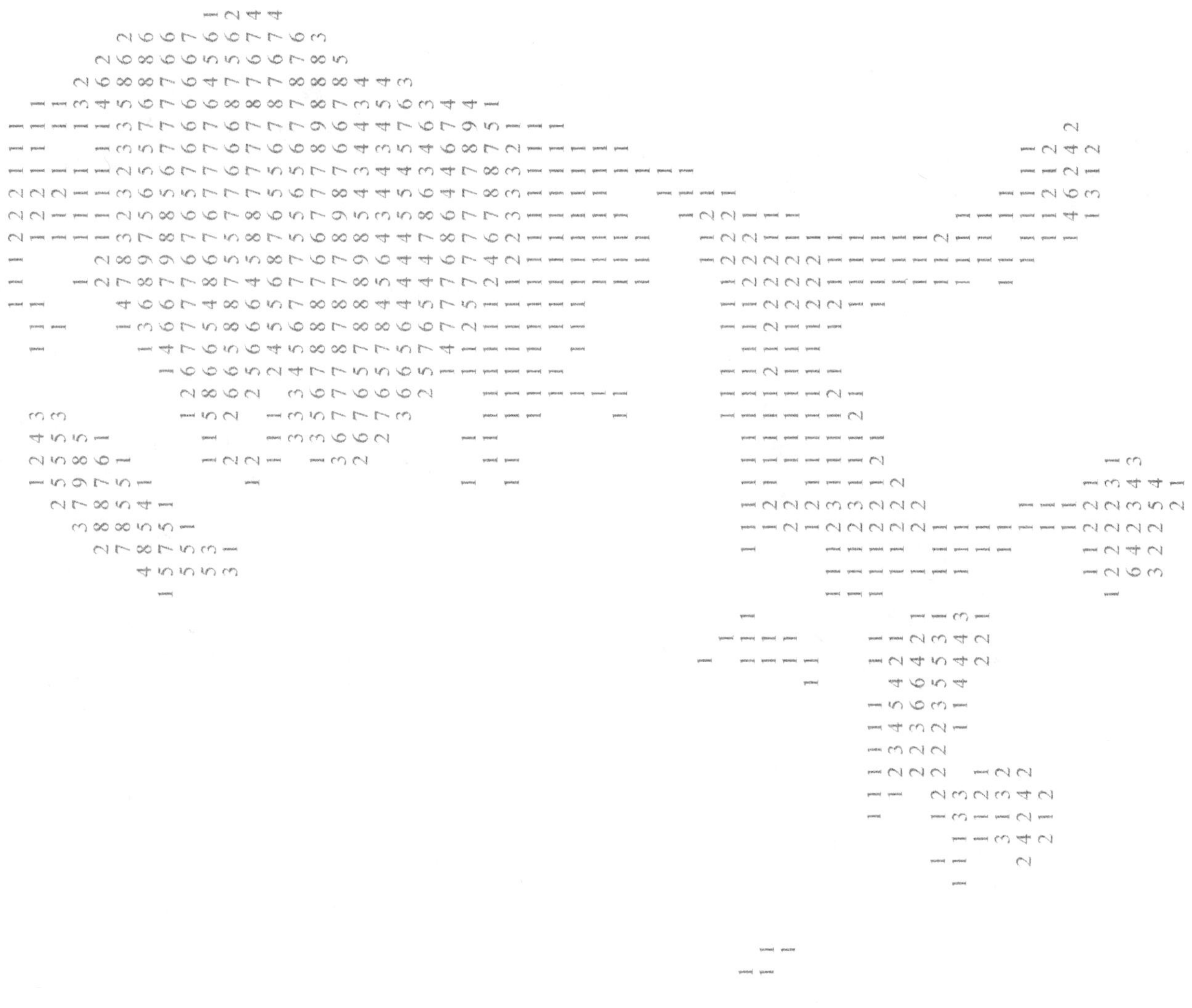

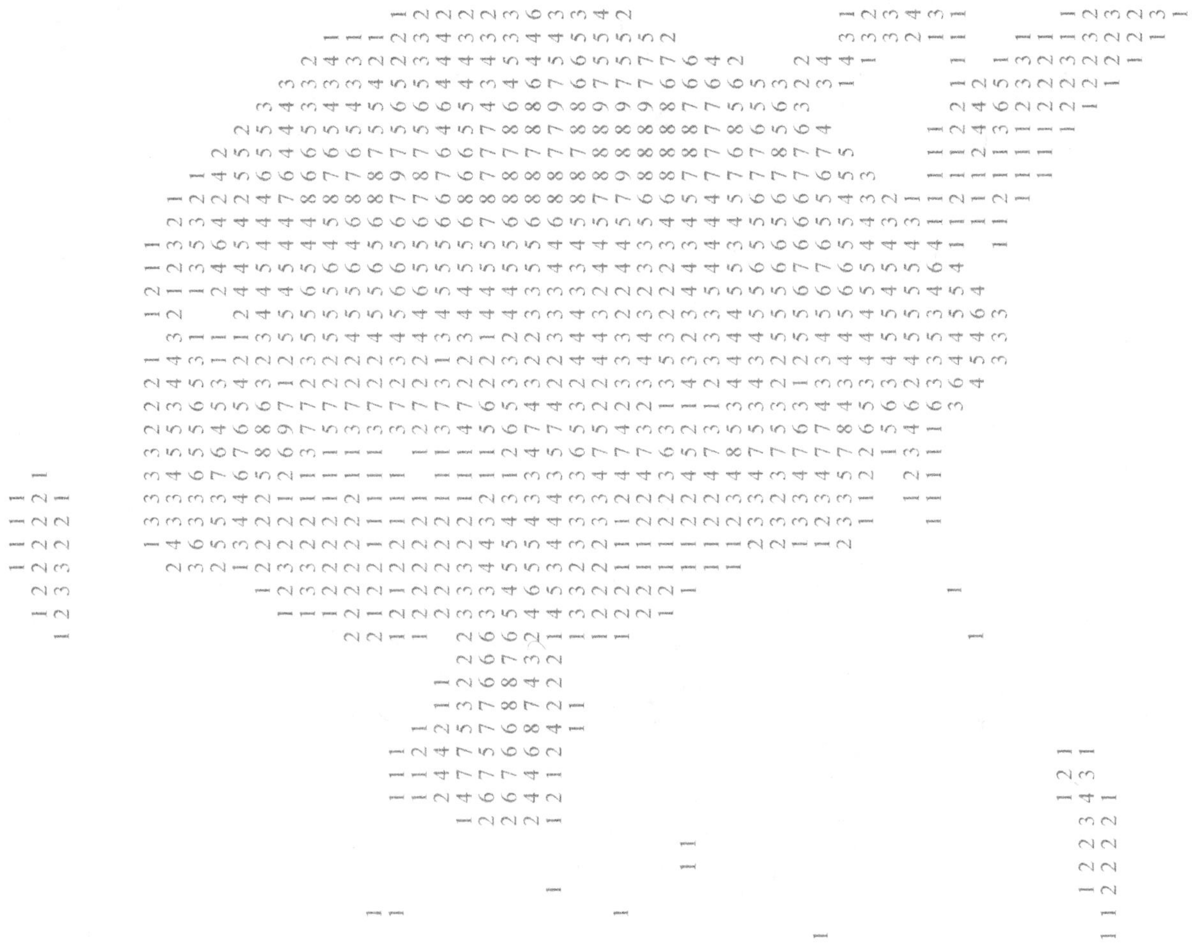

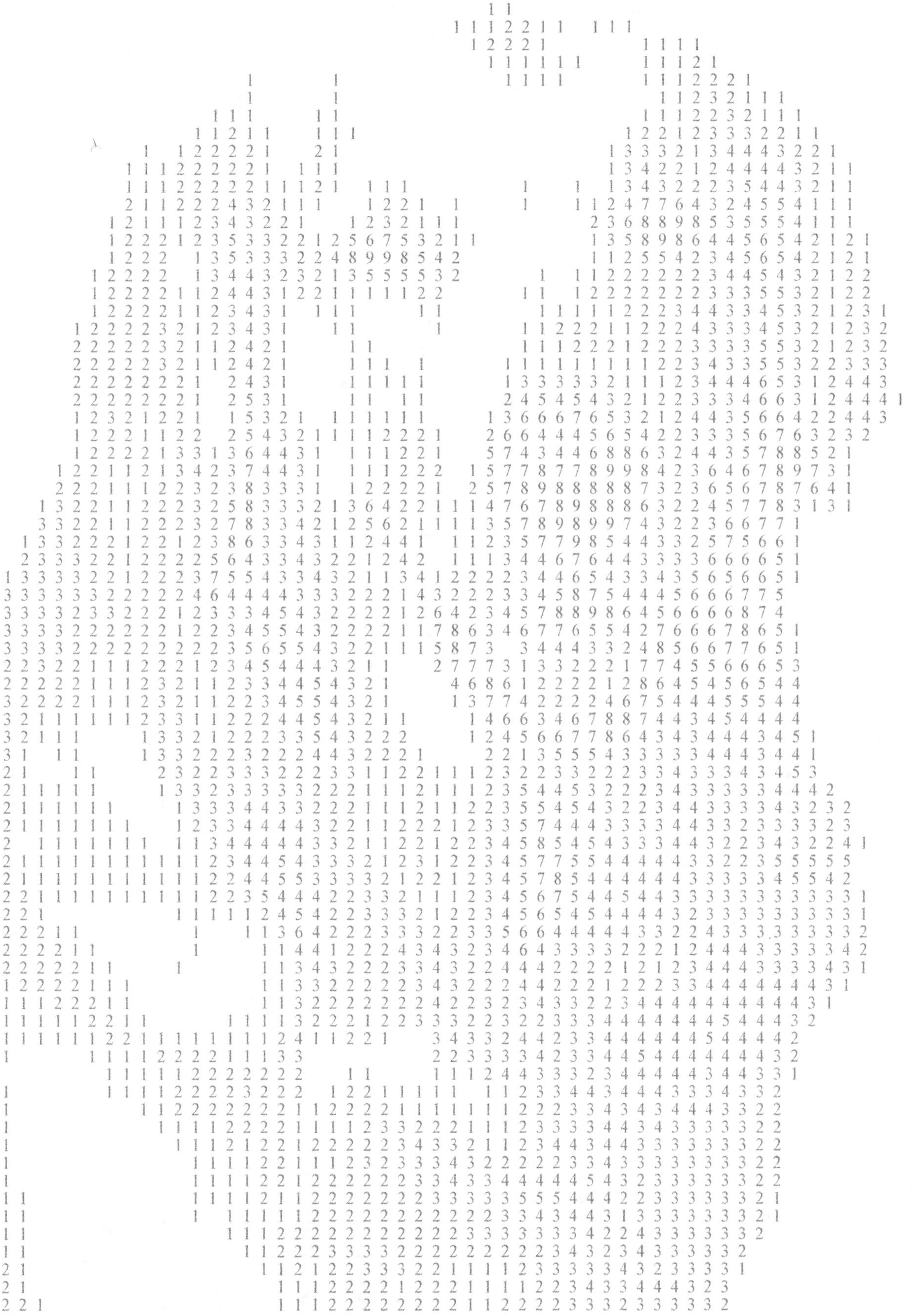

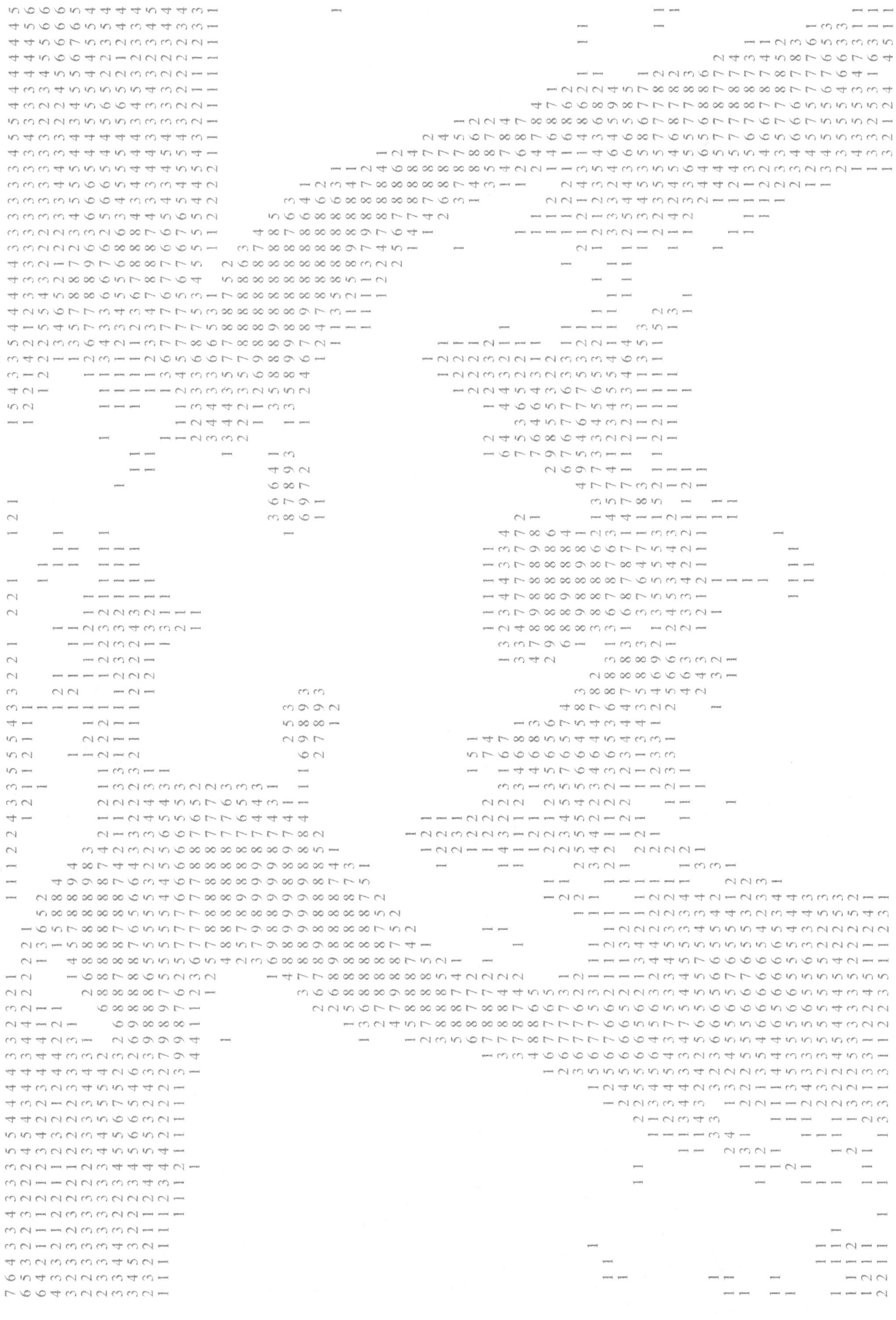

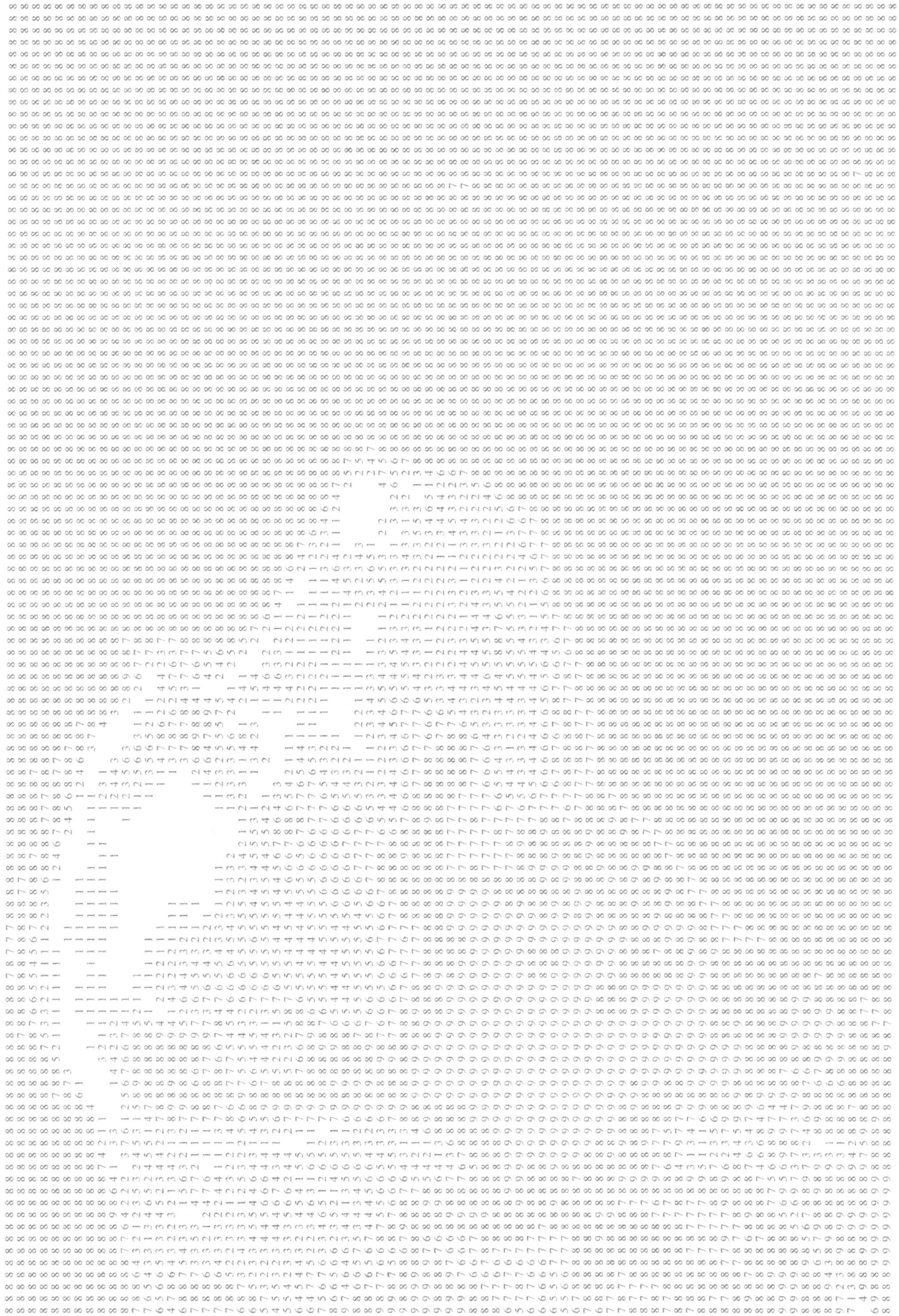

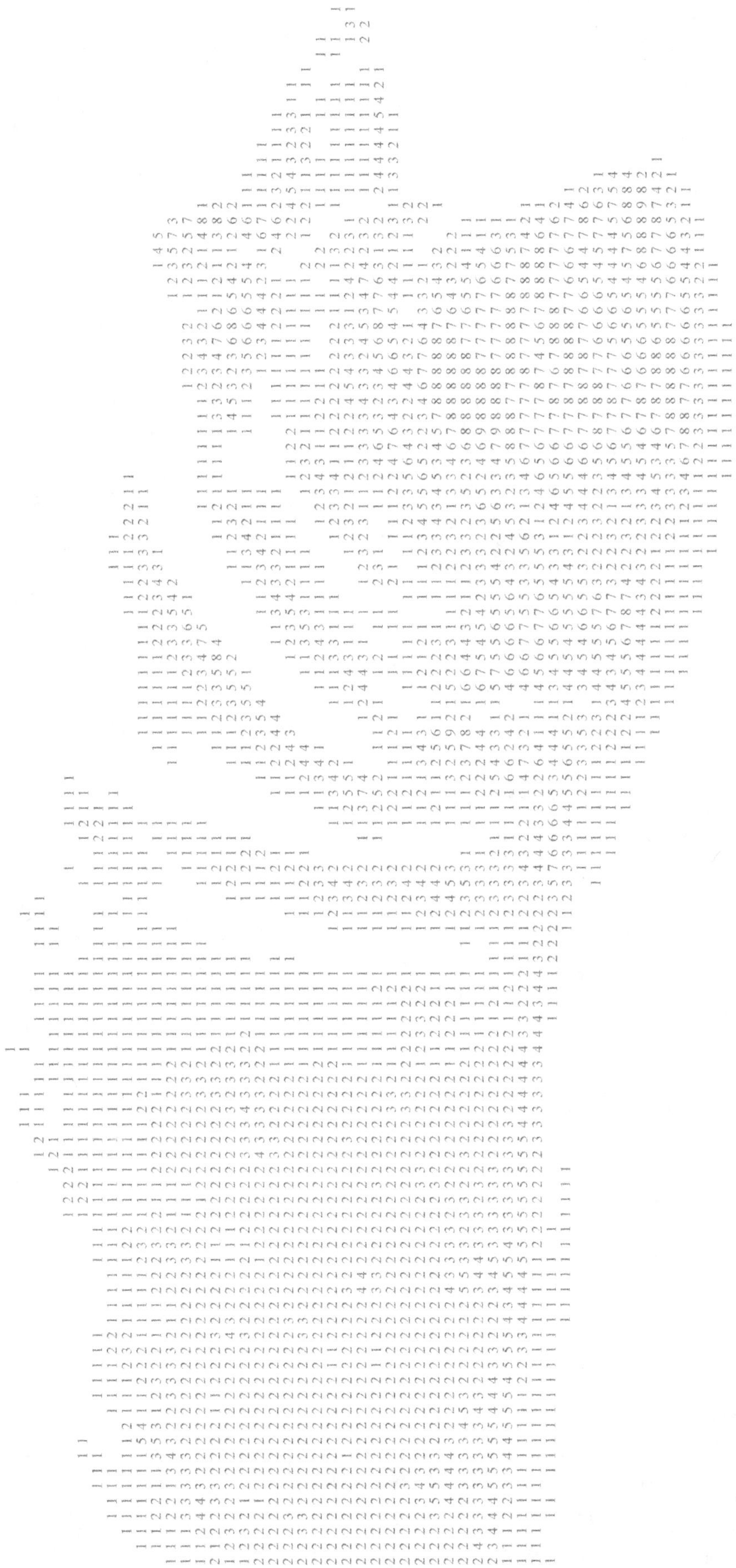

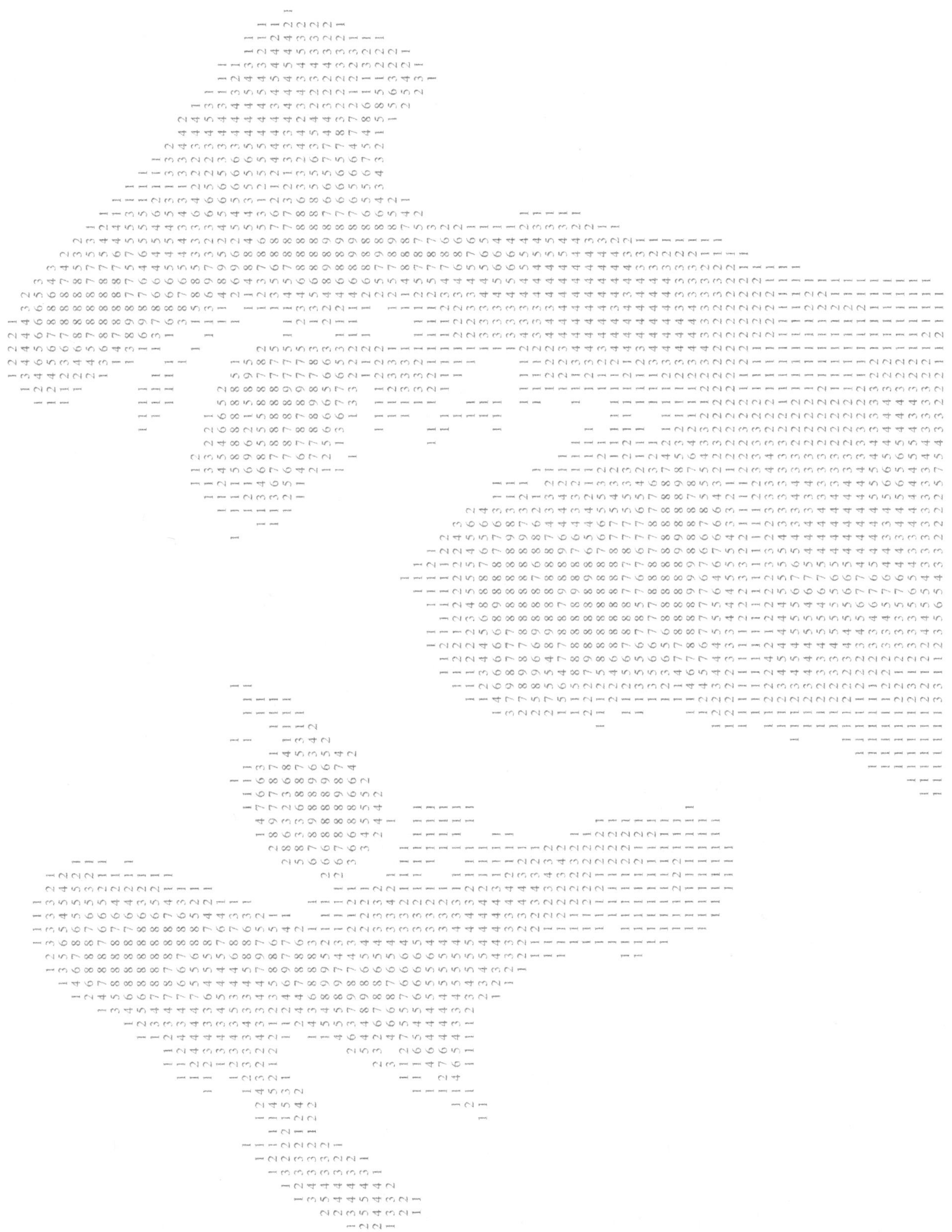

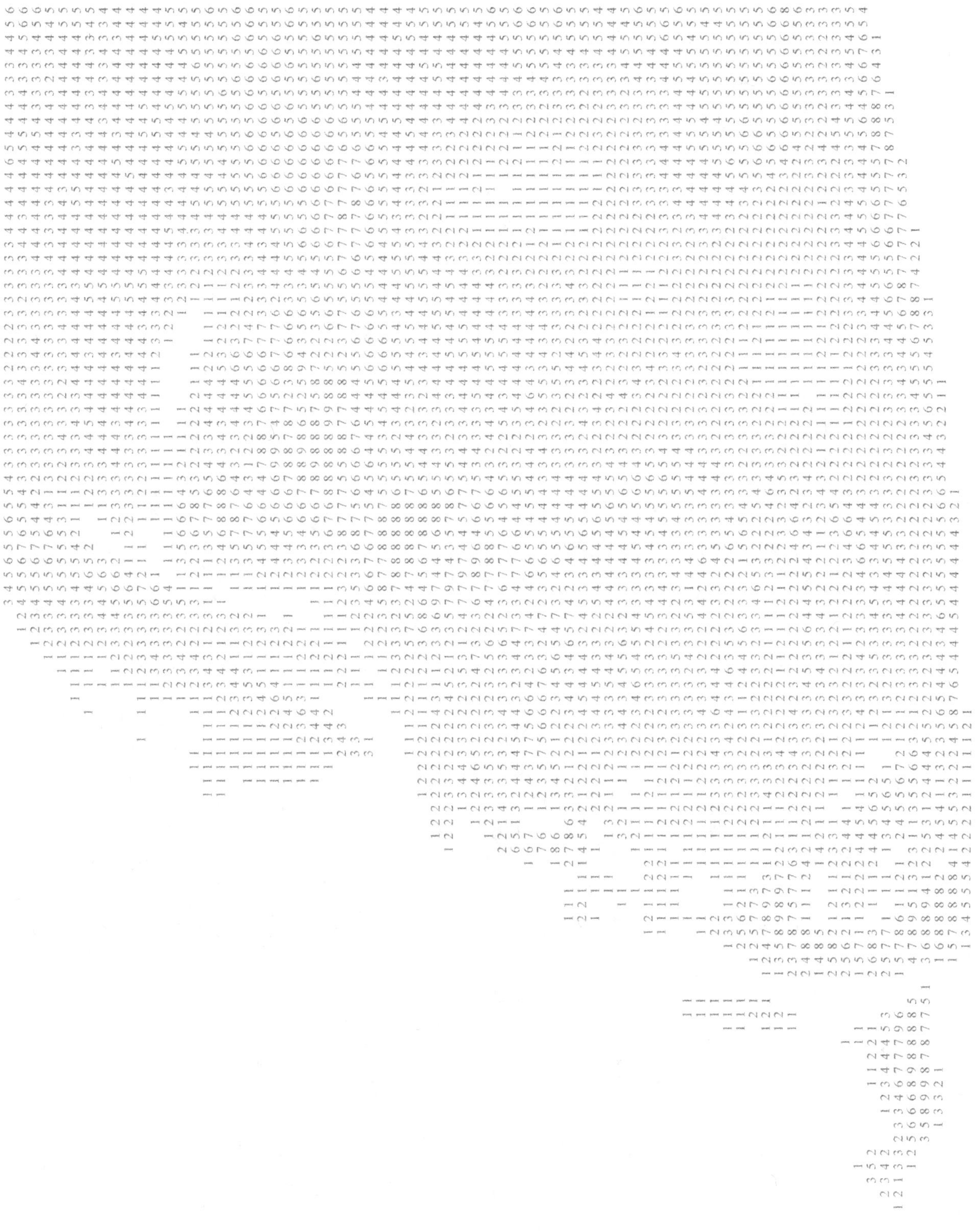

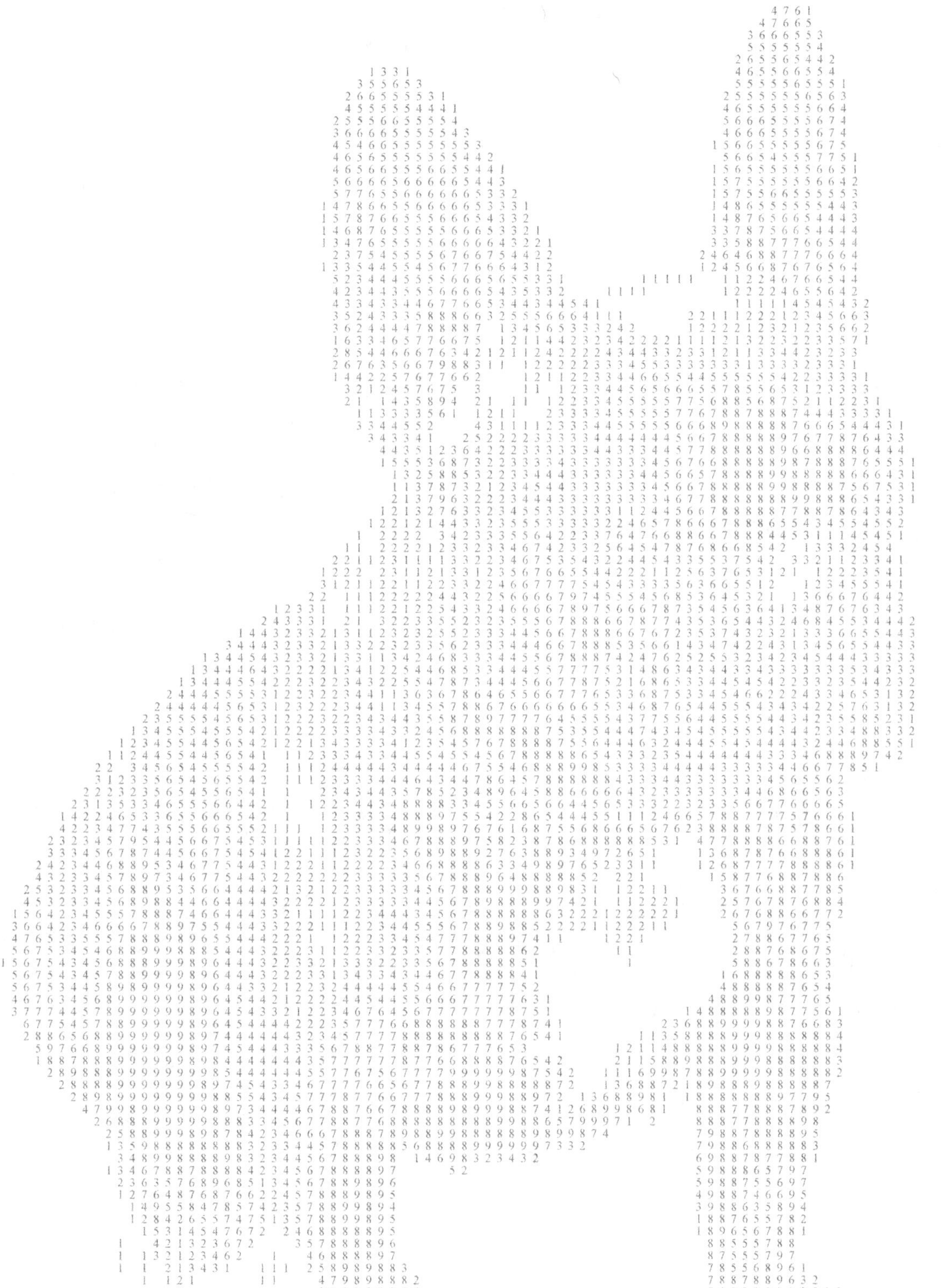

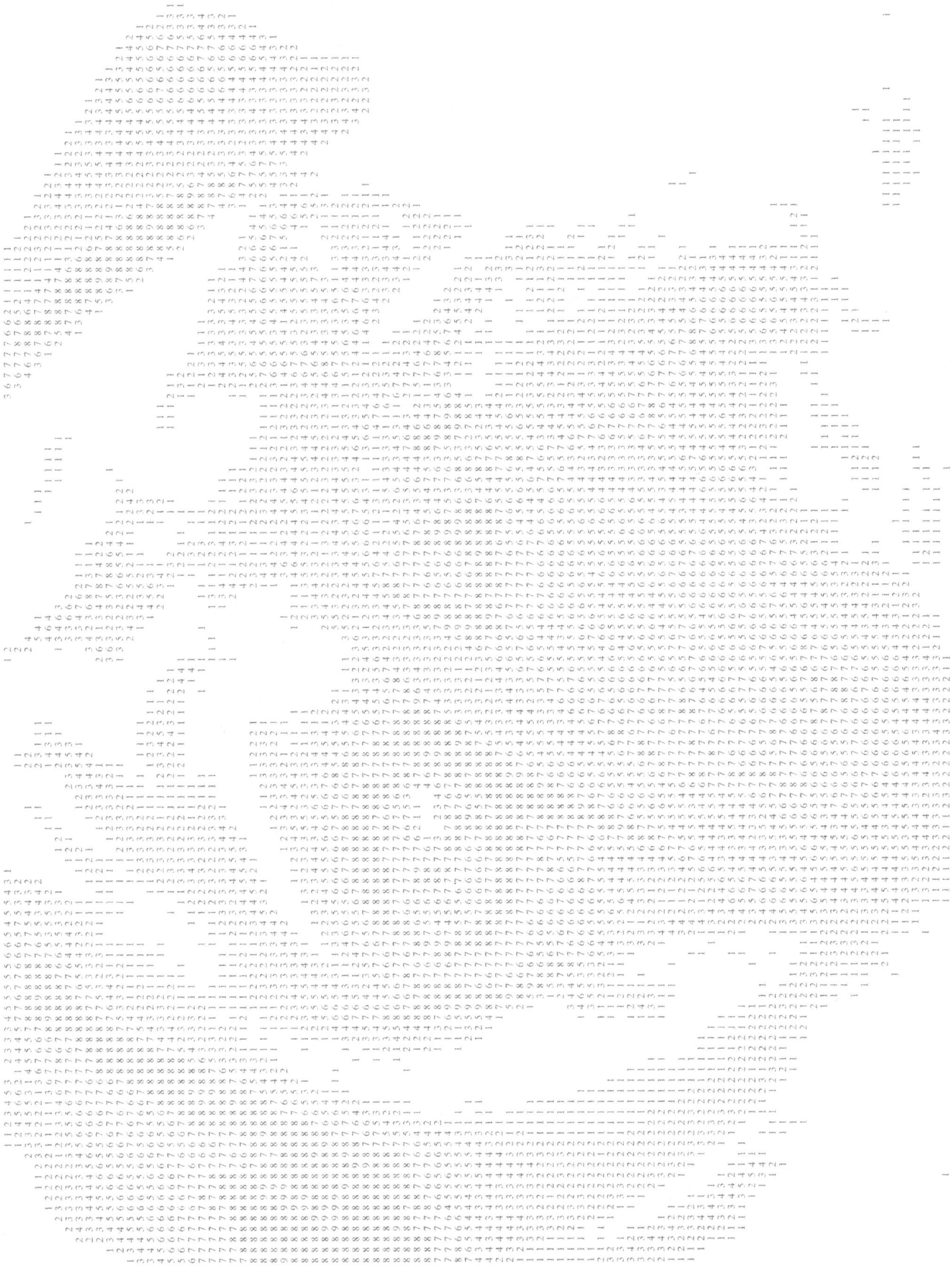

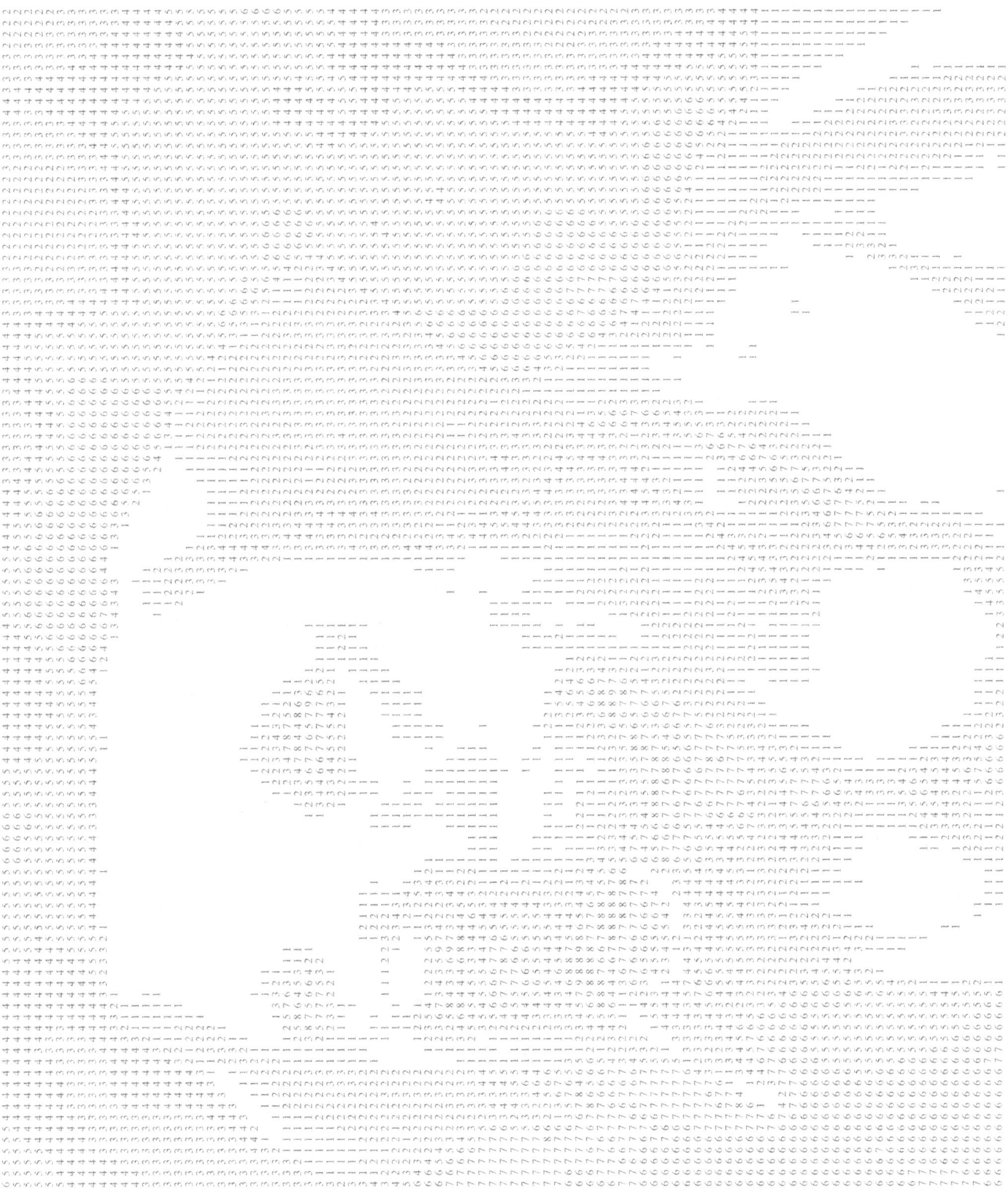

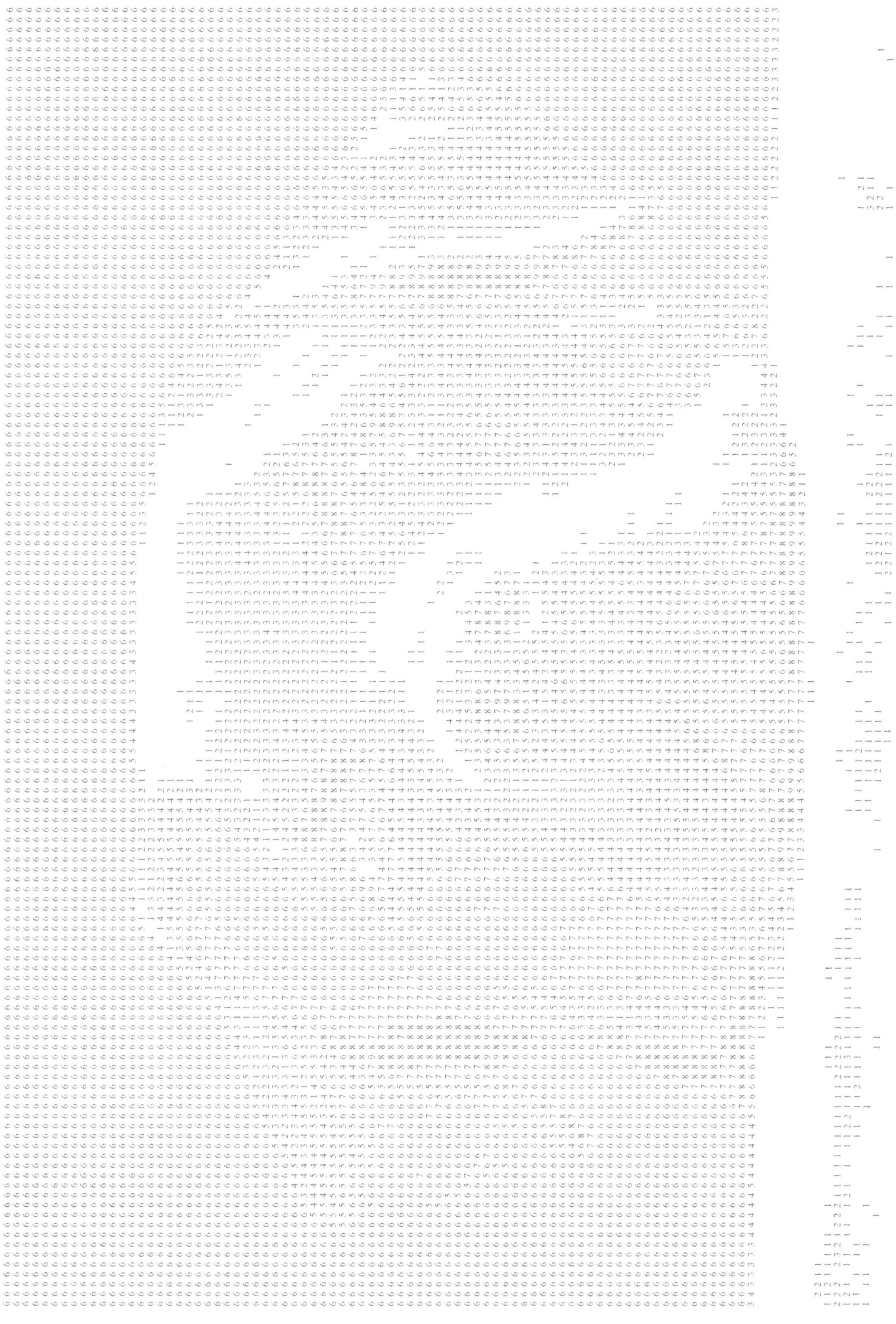

Thanks

We hope you enjoyed Dot Discovery. If you did, please leave us a review on Amazon. Reviews are a great way to let us know that you liked creating the images. We love to see samples of others work. If you share Dot Discovery on social media, please use the hashtag `#dotdiscovery`.

Dot Discovery books can help your youth, school, sports, and other groups make a great fundraiser. We have a wonderful affiliate program, using our existing books, or we can also use your images to make a custom book for your group. Visit http://dotdiscovery.com for more details.

Want More Dots?

If you just can't get enough dots, try our Dot Discovery MyDots program. Simply send an image of your choice to us, and we'll send you a custom printable version of your image so you can discover friends, family, and more! Turn any picture into an activity that everyone can enjoy. Visit http://dotdiscovery.com for more details.